Veronica Vieira
Diogo A. Rondon
Luiz A. Moscon

Dental prophylaxis in horses

Veronica Vieira
Diogo A. Rondon
Luiz A. Moscon

Dental prophylaxis in horses

Effectiveness of Equine Dental Prophylaxis in terms of Fecal Fiber Evaluation

ScienciaScripts

Imprint
Any brand names and product names mentioned in this book are subject to trademark, brand or patent protection and are trademarks or registered trademarks of their respective holders. The use of brand names, product names, common names, trade names, product descriptions etc. even without a particular marking in this work is in no way to be construed to mean that such names may be regarded as unrestricted in respect of trademark and brand protection legislation and could thus be used by anyone.

Cover image: www.ingimage.com

This book is a translation from the original published under ISBN 978-613-9-68566-0.

Publisher:
Sciencia Scripts
is a trademark of
Dodo Books Indian Ocean Ltd. and OmniScriptum S.R.L publishing group

120 High Road, East Finchley, London, N2 9ED, United Kingdom
Str. Armeneasca 28/1, office 1, Chisinau MD-2012, Republic of Moldova, Europe
Printed at: see last page
ISBN: 978-620-8-21885-0

SUMMARY

To my family, friends and teachers who helped me to persist and not give up on my dreams.

To God, for giving me strength, opportunities and accompanying me throughout my journey.

To my family, who made it possible and gave me all the support I needed to become a veterinary doctor.

My mother, who gave me encouragement and support when I needed to keep trying.

To my friends, who walked with me in the daily struggle to study and dedicate themselves to the profession, helping me in moments of despair and in the paraphrasing of my monograph.

To my teacher and advisor Diogo Rondon for guiding me all the way, from the beginning of the monograph.

I would also like to thank my colleagues Lago Tureta, Joao Victor Careta, Amanda Martins and Daniel Generoso, who encouraged me and made it possible for me to carry out my work.

To the horses for always being so perfect.

To teachers and staff.

Thank you so much!

"If we can dream, we can also make

our dreams come true."

Walt Disney

SUMMARY

Irregularities in the dental occlusion surface cause jaw movement restrictions in horses during chewing, as well as contributing to a drop in performance during exercise due to oral pain. In order to identify which dental wear alterations most affect animals that have never undergone dental treatment and to prove the effectiveness of dental prophylaxis by measuring the size of the animals' fecal fibers, 30 horses were evaluated and the main dental alterations found in the horses were: excessive tooth enamel tips (100%), ramp (13.33%), flattening (10%), rostral hook (20%), swallow tail (23.33%) , ulcer (23.33%), wolf tooth (20%) and wave (6.66%). In the fecal fiber evaluation, there was a decline of 1cm on average per animal. Based on the results, it can be seen that dental prophylaxis in horses creates comfort for the animal when feeding and improves intestinal transit, which will consequently reduce gastrointestinal problems.

Keywords: Dentistry, dental disorders, equine.

INTRODUCTION

The increasingly early domestication and confinement of animals has favored the modification of eating habits and patterns, thus compromising natural dental formation and leading to a series of dental disorders.

Dental problems often cause intra-oral lacerations in the soft tissues, causing pain when chewing, a change in biomechanics, a drop in performance and a change in the fecal bolus. Some oral disorders are diagnosed late.

In these situations, chronic weight loss in horses is related to dental disorders. Most of these alterations can be corrected and contribute to the increased breakdown of fiber and nutrients in the equine diet, even in those without oral lesions and with an adequate body score.

After the prophylaxis has been carried out, some precautions are necessary to avoid complications in the post-procedure period. Immediate fasting should be observed, and after sedation with Detomidine Hydrochloride, non-steroidal anti-inflammatory drugs should be used to control any inflammatory processes that may occur, such as pain, edema, heat, redness and loss of tissue function. If there is damage at the time of prophylaxis, antibiotics can be used prophylactically.

In order to reduce these alterations, equine clinical practice has increasingly emphasized the importance of dentistry. This area of equine medicine studies and treats the horse's entire stomatognathic system.

An experimental study was carried out on a farm chosen for the study, located in the municipality of Linhares - ES and on a property in Colatina -ES. The faeces collected from the selected horses were processed and analyzed in the chemistry laboratory of the Centro Universitàrio do Espirito Santo - UNESC, which provided the relevant data for the study.

Therefore, this study aimed to evaluate the effectiveness of dental prophylaxis in horses by measuring the fibers in the feces and their importance in animal welfare and health. Since the results were very satisfactory for the first dental treatment of each animal, on average we obtained a drop of 0.58 cm in fecal fibers. We can therefore affirm the effectiveness of dental treatment in horses, generating comfort when feeding and improving intestinal transit, which will consequently reduce gastrointestinal problems.

1 OBJECTIVES

1.108   GENERAL OBJECTIVES

To evaluate the different changes in the parameters studied, in order to demonstrate the benefits of dental treatments in horses.

1.109   SPECIFIC OBJECTIVES

> To evaluate the changes generated in the animal's posture before and after dental prophylaxis.

> Measure the amount of fiber contained in the feces of horses before and after dental prophylaxis.

> Compare the animal's physical performance before and after dental prophylaxis.

2 THEORETICAL FRAMEWORK

Equine dentistry has been practiced for centuries, with the oldest record dating back to 1207 AD, the first book published in this field dates back to 1889, and was written by T D Hinebauch, professor of Veterinary Sciences at Purdue University, and the first equine dentistry school was opened in 1980 in Glenns Ferry, Idaho (SILVA et al., 2003).

Brazil has the second largest equine herd in the world, with approximately seven million animals. However, the number of animals receiving any kind of dental care is very low. It is well known that good oral health must be established in order to keep horses healthy, since digestive problems are the main cause of illness in these animals (ALVES, 2004).

Veterinary dentistry is known to be a field of study in full development. Today, it is believed and defended that preventive dental care denotes zeal for property (ALVES, 2004). In horses, dentistry has proved to be an important tool for ensuring a good quality of life, maintaining health and improving sporting function. Dental corrections should be carried out periodically (BOTELHO *et al.*, 2007), avoiding the development of serious anomalies or slowing down progress (DIXON and DU TOIT, 2012; RALSTON *et al.*, 2001).

It is important to include an examination of the oral cavity in the clinical examination of foals soon after birth, so that congenital problems can be diagnosed quickly and the necessary measures can be taken. The presence of any palate or lip defects, symmetry of the head and masticatory function should be observed, as well as assessing the sequence of tooth eruption, including the alignment of the incisors. When there is a disparity between the incisor teeth, the unequal alignment of the molars and premolars can lead to rostral hooks on the second premolars and caudal hooks on the third molars (DACRE and DIXON, 2005).

Good dental practice requires periodic, biannual inspections that allow for a timely diagnosis of any changes and the prevention of their impact on the equine's clinical state (BOTELHO *et al.*, 2007).

2.1 anatomical and physiological characteristics

Like other domestic mammals, the horse's teeth are classified as heterodonts, i.e. they are made up of different types or groups of teeth - incisors, canines, premolars and molars - each of which has specific characteristics and functions, with the incisors cutting, the canines holding and tearing, and the premolars and molars crushing and grinding food (DIXON, 1999).

In horses, "the space between the canines and the premolars present in an arch is called a bar or diastema and is particularly large when the canines are absent" (SILVA et al., 2003), which is especially the case in females.

The entrance to the digestive tract is formed by strong and extremely mobile lips. The horse grasps food mainly with its lips and tongue, and when grazing or eating firmer substances (branches and tubers) the incisors (upper and lower) are also used, allowing it to graze close to the ground, cutting the forage. The upper lip is used to place the forage between the horse's teeth (MEYER,

1997; FRAPE, 2008).

Saliva is only produced and mixed with food during chewing. Therefore, the time of ingestion has a great influence on this factor. Horses produce around 40-90 ml of saliva per minute, an amount that varies according to the nature of the food (FRAPE, 2008).

Since horses have two sets of teeth, the first being deciduous, temporary or milk, and the second, permanent or definitive, these animals are also classified as diphiodonts (SILVA et al., 2003) **(Figure 1)**.

Figure 1 Schematic representation of the four different groups of equine teeth

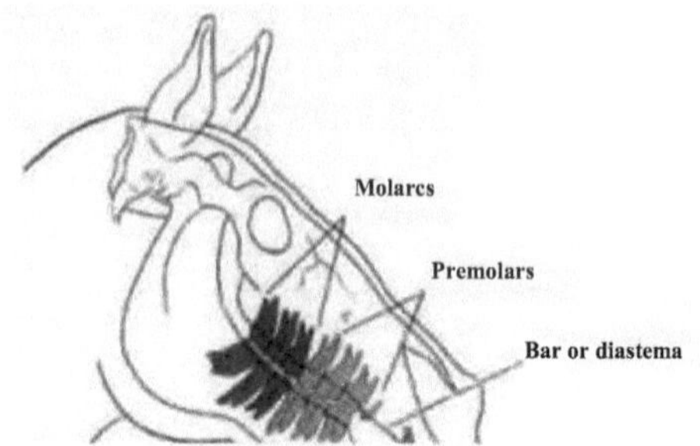

Source: Adapted from KRELING (2003).

It is known that horses' teeth grow by 0.3 to 0.4 cm a year, which means that by the end of the year the upper and lower teeth have grown by almost a centimeter, but thanks to the wear and tear that occurs every day from chewing, the teeth always remain at their normal size (BREDER, 2010).

Equine teeth have long crowns, from seven to ten centimeters in the apico-coronal direction, and are classified as hypsodonts. The visible portion of a tooth element in the oral cavity is called the clinical crown and the portion inserted into the dental socket is made up of the reserve crown and roots. Dentin, enamel and cementum on the occlusal surface are constantly remodeled thanks to the difference in resistance between the three tissues that make up teeth (LOWDER; MUELLER, 1998).

Inside the tooth is the pulp cavity, the shape of which resembles the tooth. In the root, this cavity ends in a hole called the apical foramen, through which the vessels and nerves that supply the tooth pass (CARNEIRO and JUNQUEIRA,

1995; SILVA et al., 2003).

The pulp, an innervated and highly vascularized connective tissue that constitutes the internal structure of the tooth, is found in the pulp cavity or chamber (SILVA et al., 2003).

According to DACRE (2006), around two to six millimeters (mm) of secondary dentin are deposited between the occlusal surface of pre-molars (with the exception of the first) and molars and their pulp.

The periodontium, the name given to the structures responsible for fixing teeth, includes the cementum, the periodontal ligament and the alveolar bone (SILVA et al., 2003).

The cementum, a specialized mineralized tissue, covers the tooth root (CARNEIRO and JUNQUEIRA, 1995; SILVA et al., 2003) **(Figure 2)**.

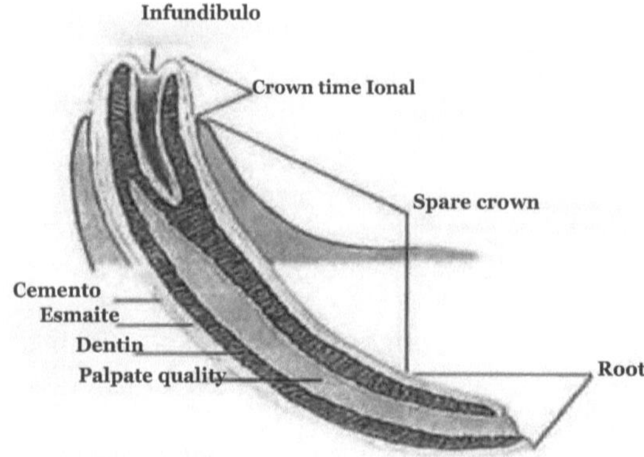

Figure 2 **Anatomy of an equine incisor tooth.**

Source: Adapted from LOWDER and MUELLER (1998).

Equines have twelve (12) incisor teeth, six of which are mandibular incisors and six maxillary incisors. The incisor teeth have the function of grasping and cutting forage. Horses that are confined and do not have access to grazing do not use their incisor teeth to cut forage and this can make these teeth much longer than the normal pattern, due to the lack of friction (EASLEY, 1996).

The canine teeth are usually located in the diastema of adult males. They almost always erupt between 4.5 and 6 years of age, which corresponds to the beginning of peak sexual maturity. It is believed that their function is to defend the herd and fight other males. The upper canines are located at the junction of the lateral incisors and the upper canines. Together with the lower incisors, the lower canines support the tongue in the relaxed horse. When present in mares, the canines are vestigial, mainly in the mandible (EASLEY, 2004).

12

The lobe teeth are the first vestigial premolars and occur inconsistently (DACRE and DIXON, 2005). These lobe teeth may be absent or rudimentary (LOWDER and MUELLER, 1998).

The adult equine has 12 premolar and 12 molar teeth, which form 4 rows of 6 teeth accommodated in the mandible and maxilla bones (EASLEY, 2006; LOWDER and MUELLER, 1998; DIXON, 2005). Their function is to grind and chew food when the main physical-mechanical phenomena of digestion occur. The importance of these phenomena is to initiate the digestive process in the mouth and create the conditions for the other subsequent digestive processes to take place (ALVES, 2004).

Dental alterations can affect the biomechanics of the masticatory cycle and impair the proper grinding of food (BAKER, 2002) **(Figure 3)**.

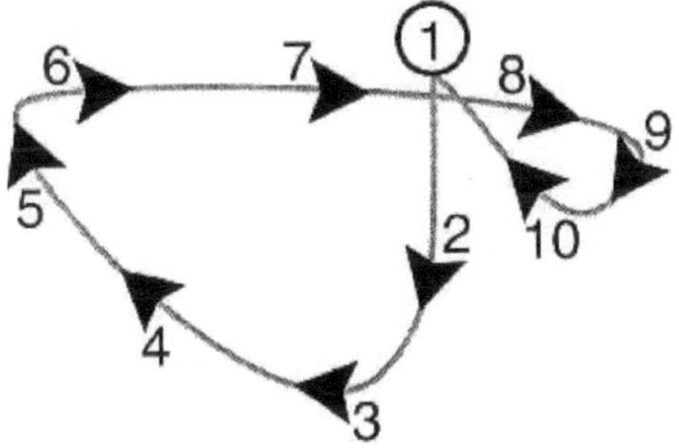

Figura 2   **Diagram of the phases of the equine masticatory cycle defined according to mandibular movement, represented by the continuous line. The numbers from 1 to 3 represent the opening phase; 4 and 5, the closing phase; from 6 to 9, the impact and friction (IA) phase; and the**

Source: Adapted from BAKER (2002).

The equine dental formula for deciduous teeth is: 2 x (incisors 3/3, canines

0/0, premolars 3/3 and molars 0/0). For permanent teeth: 2 x (incisors 3/3, canines 1/1 (males), or 0/0 (females), premolars 3/3 or 4/4 and molars 3/3) = 36 to 44 teeth, depending on the presence and quantity of wolf teeth and canines (DIXON, 2005; TOIT, 2006).

2 (Di 3/3, Dc 0/0, Dpm 3/3) = 24 dentes	2 (I3/3, C1/1 ou 0/0, PM 3/3 ou 4/4, M 3/3)

2.1.1 Classification of the dental arch

Two systems are used to identify a tooth in the equine: an anatomical system and a numerical system. The anatomical system names the tooth according to its function (e.g. incisors and pre-molars). The numerical system, known as the Modified Triadan System, identifies each tooth with a particular number. Knowledge of timing and eruption is important for understanding both systems (LOWDER,1998).

In the anatomical system, the type of tooth to be described is defined by a letter, with deciduous teeth represented by lower case letters (i = incisors, p = premolars) and permanent teeth by upper case letters (I = incisors, C = canines, P = premolars, M = molars). To this letter is then attached a number that defines the location of the tooth in the oral cavity, which is admittedly divided into four quadrants, the right side of the maxillary arch being considered the first, followed by the others (second, third and fourth), in clockwise order. The location of the tooth is then represented by the letter and the 8 number around it, thus positioning it in one of the four quadrants (e.g. 1I = first permanent right incisor of the mandibular arch;[3] M = third permanent right molar of the maxillary arch; p^2 = second temporary left premolar of the maxillary arch; i3 = third temporary left incisor of the mandibular arch). This system has gradually fallen into disuse (LOWDER, 1998; FOSTER, 2008) **(Figure 4)**.

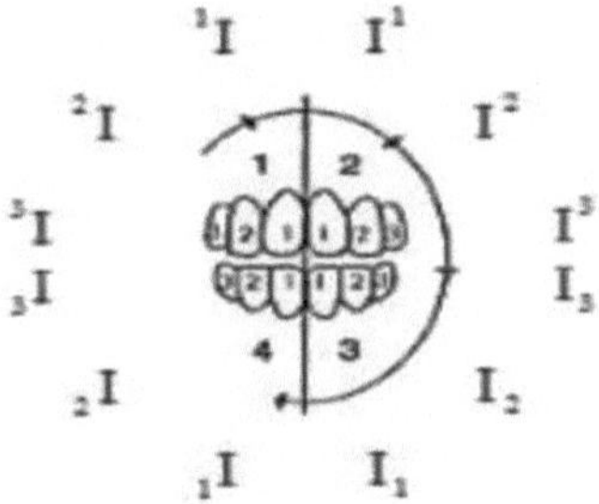

Figura 4   **Representative diagram of the anatomical system for permanent incisor teeth.**

Source: Adapted from FOSTER (2008).

In the modified Triadan system, which is an exclusively numerical system, each tooth is described by three digits. The first refers to the quadrant, with permanent teeth numbered from 1 to 4 (clockwise), and deciduous teeth from 5 to 8. For example: 1 identifies the upper right quadrant of permanent teeth, 7 identifies the lower left quadrant of deciduous teeth. The second and third digits of this nomenclature identify the tooth within the respective quadrant (e.g. 1 identifies the first incisor and 11 the last molar). For a better understanding and as an example: the number 311 identifies the last permanent left molar of the lower arch, the number 108 identifies the fourth permanent right premolar of the upper arch, the number 601 refers to the first deciduous left incisor of the upper arch, the number 806 indicates the second deciduous right premolar of the lower arch. (DIXON, 1999).

This system is currently the most widely used (LOWDER, 1998) **(Figure 5)**.

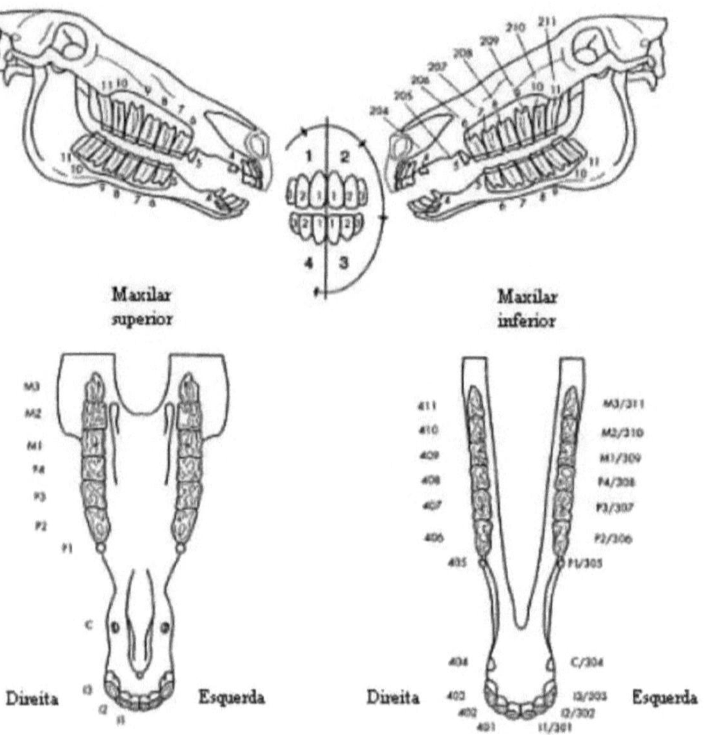

Figura 5   **Schematic representation of the modified Triadan system for permanent teeth**

Source: Adapted from FOSTER (2008).

2.2 DENTAL PROPHYLAXIS

Of the oral diseases that affect horses, dental occurrences are the most important in equine veterinary practice. They constitute the third most common case in the abundant animal practice in the United States. In addition, post-mortem studies have shown significant findings of undiagnosed dental problems in horses (DACRE and DIXON, 2005).

Equine dental examinations should be carried out twice a year, as part of the animal's routine health maintenance program (SMITH, 2006).

Routine dental care is essential for equine health. Periodic examinations and regular maintenance are extremely necessary due to the changes in equine diet and eating patterns that have occurred mainly with the advent of domestication and confinement of these animals. All of this together greatly alters the natural wear and maintenance of the teeth (SOUZA, 2009).

2.3 INSPECTION OF THE ORAL CAVITY

The repercussions of dental alterations on the animal's conformation and performance are often underestimated. However, it is known that a regular examination of the oral cavity, particularly the teeth, preferably biannually, is considered sufficient to prevent these alterations and/or identify them early, thus enabling timely treatment before any complications arise (BAKER, 2002).

A good dental inspection should be carried out in a certain order, starting with a previous history, followed by an external inspection of the horse, checking the mobility of the head and jaw and only lastly an internal inspection of the oral cavity without a mouth opener and with a mouth opener (ALVES,2004).

External inspection can be carried out in three stages: visual, olfactory and tactile. During the visual inspection, special attention should be paid to the general condition of the animal, the symmetry, conformation and shape of the head, the presence of inflammations, deformations, abscesses in the mandible and maxilla or possible nasal discharge; the symmetry of the temporo-mandibular joints, among others. The olfactory inspection checks for the presence of halitosis, which can be indicative of oral pathology. In the tactile inspection phase, the premolar and molar areas, the temporo-mandibular joints, the space between the mandible and the wings of the atlas, the head ganglia and salivary glands should be palpated externally. Any alterations, deformations or painful areas on palpation should be looked for (MANSO and SAN ROMAN, 2002).

2.3.1 Materials used for oral inspection

Due to the wide variety of alterations that can be found in the mouth of an equine, the increased demand for dental services in this species and also due to the increased use of sedatives and analgesics that allow for better restraint of the animal, a wide range of instruments has been developed with the aim of improving the quantity and quality of dental practice in horses. The choice of instruments varies according to the pathology present, the veterinarian's knowledge, experience and personal tastes, and must meet the requirements of ease of handling, comfort of use and guarantee of good results (EASLEY, 1998).

The equipment used to carry out dental prophylaxis can be of two types:

manual and electric (THOMASSIAN, 2005).

The most commonly used dental instruments for good inspection and treatment are: Mouth opener, photophore, syringe or pump, mirror, goggles, apical levers, manual and electric coarse levers (ALVES, 2004), **(Figures 6, 7, 8, 9, 10, 11, 12)**.

Mouth opener

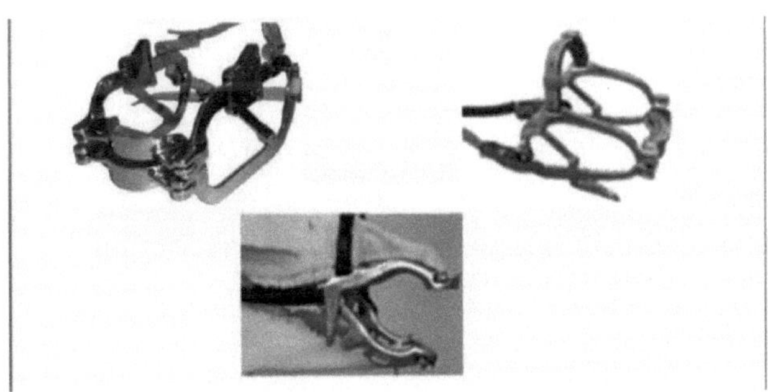

Figure 6 : **McPherson opener**

Source:

http://www.dentistadecavalo.com.br/images/stories/abridor%20de%

20boca.jpg. Accessed on November 20, 2014.

Hand-operated rasps

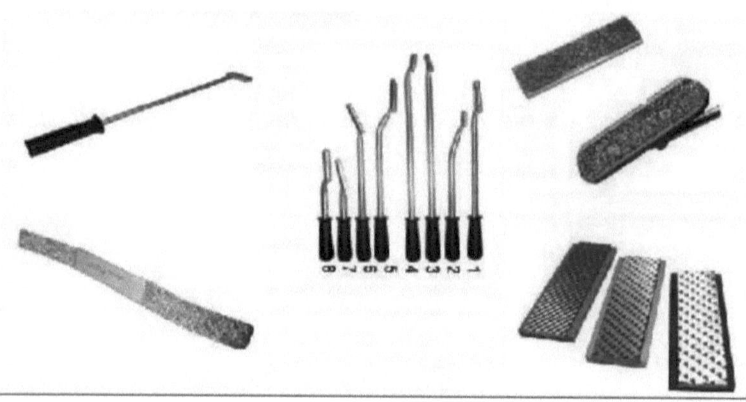

Source:

http://www.dentistadecavalo.com.br/images/stories/grosas%20man

uais.jpg. Accessed on Nov. 20, 2014.

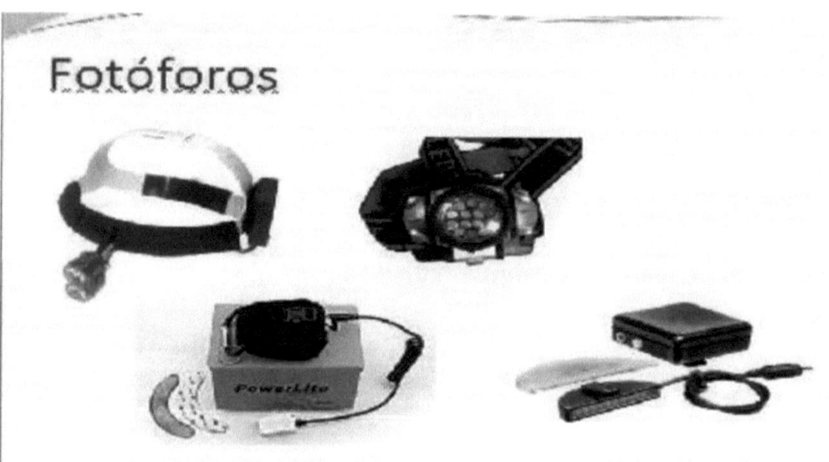

Figura 8: **Photophores**

Source:

http://www.dentistadecavalo.com.br/images/stories/fotoforos.jpg.

Accessed on Nov. 20, 2014.

Apóío for dental head & headgear

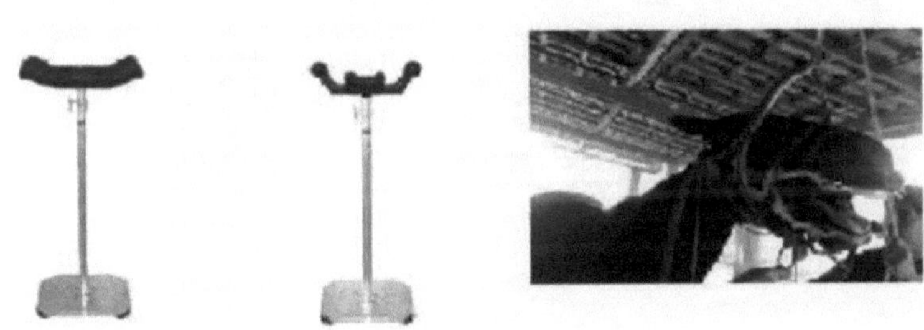

Figura 9:   Headrest.

Source:

http://www.dentistadecavalo.com.br/images/stories/cabeada%20od

ontologica.jpg.Accessed on 20 Nov. 2014.

Levers, pliers, apothecaries, etc.

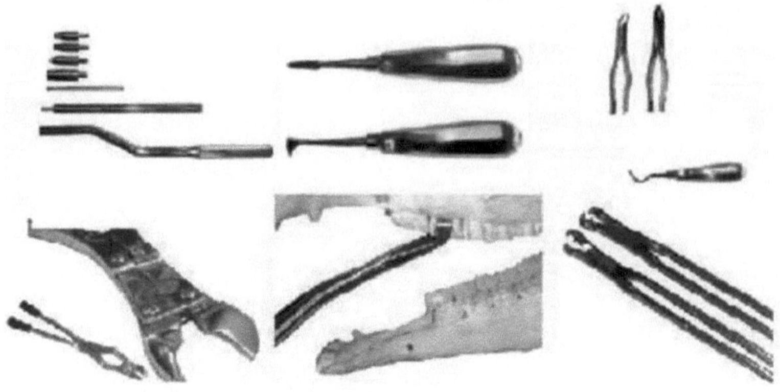

Figure 10: Levers, pliers and buttons.

Source:

http://www.dentistadecavalo.com.br/images/stories/alavancas.jpg.

Accessed on Nov. 20, 2014.

Glasses, syringes and pump.

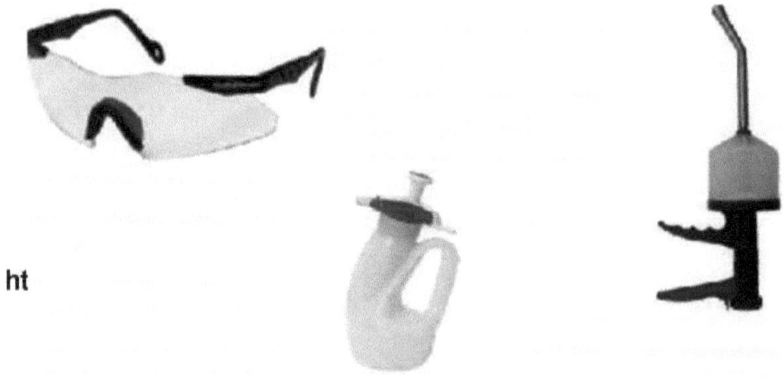

ht

Figure 11: Eyepiece, syringe and pump.

Source:

http://www.dentistadecavalo.com.br/images/stories/oculos.jpg.

Accessed on Nov. 20, 2014.

2.4 MAIN DENTAL CONDITIONS

Some dental pathologies can be the result of various etiologies, making it very difficult to define the actual agent(s) that triggered the pathological process (BAKER, 2002).

2.4.1 Fractures

Malocclusion causes tooth fractures and the formation of sharp surfaces that can injure the tongue and cheek and cause very painful ulcers (MANsO and SAN ROMaN, 2002).

A high incidence of sagittal palatal, lingual and vestibular dental fractures and proximal and distal mesial fractures is observed at sites of marked iatrogenic prematurity. In chronic processes, extrusion of the antagonist occlusal surface can displace the premature contact point to the opposite hemiface, predisposing the region to new dental fractures. Old fractures of the first or second molar teeth are frequently observed, causing such intense occlusal disharmony that fractures occur in a similar region on the other side of the arch. Teeth with cemental hypoplasia are more likely to fracture as a result of occlusal trauma. The compaction of food at fracture sites favors the development of periodontal disease (SOUZA, 2009).

The most commonly used osteosynthesis technique for maxillary and mandibular fractures is cerclage on adjacent teeth. In more extensive and unstable fractures, cerclage can be associated with traction in a caudal direction, with support between the second and third premolars or on the canine teeth or mandibular perforation, forming a tension band (DART and PAsCOE, 1987).

2.4.2 Swallowtail

It consists of an edge, formed at the corners (incisors), due to wear of the tooth, in its most central part, so that it has a beak at the end furthest from the claws. The swallowtail appears around the age of 7 and again around the age of 13. In both cases it eventually disappears with time and even wear. During this phase, special attention should be paid to the animal's feces, trying to see if the dental situation allows it to grind and crush food well, which is vital to avoid serious problems (THOMASSIAN, 2005).

2.4.3 Lower Projection

It consists of the abnormal shortening of the mandible in relation to the pre-maxilla, without occlusion between the incisor teeth; in other words, the maxillary incisors are projected ahead of the mandibular incisor teeth (DIXON, 2005).

The main difficulties faced by those affected are pressing down on the grass in low pastures and poor chewing (ALVES, 2005).

2.4.4 Top projection

These problems occur when the incisor teeth do not touch. Upper prognathism occurs when the upper incisor teeth are in front of the lower incisors, so the animal is a lower incisor braggart, and lower prognathism occurs when the lower incisors are in front of the upper incisors, When one of these two problems occurs, the animal does not use the friction of the teeth to chew, but rather the palate (upper prognathism) or the soft part near the tongue, forming calluses in these places (lower prognathism), since the incisor teeth have no friction (DART and PASCOE, 1987).

2.4.5 Excessive nail polish tips

During chewing, enamel points appear, caused by poor occlusion of the dental arches, which can cause wounds on the cheeks and tongue, making the animal uncomfortable with the pain. Horses with enamel tips grind their food poorly, digest it slowly, lose weight progressively and are also predisposed to a high incidence of colic (THOMAZIAN, 2005).

2.4.6 Wounds

Dental alterations can cause damage to soft tissues, impairing chewing and animal performance (ALVES, 2004).

The oral mucosa should be intact, moist, covered in saliva, painless and pink in color. The presence of petechiae, hemorrhages, neoplasms or other lesions is indicative of oral pathology. The lips and tongue should be observed for shape and mobility (MANSO and SAN ROMAN , 2002).

2.4.7   Wolf's tooth

The Wolf's Tooth is a vestigial tooth and has no chewing function, but when it comes into contact with the bridle or muzzle it causes pain and discomfort in the animal. Behavioral changes while riding, such as pulling on the reins or lowering and raising the head, aggression and rebelliousness, can be mistaken for temperament problems, but are actually related to dental problems. In addition to behavioral changes, horses with disorders in the oral cavity may also show weight loss or difficulty gaining weight, accumulation of food in the mouth, slow chewing, edema of the face and/or jaw, fistulas, nasal discharge, and intestinal colic (EASLEY, 2005).

2.4.8   Tooth wear in the form of hooks and ramps

Hooks and ramps are defined as projections of the teeth by more than 1/3 of the occlusal surface. Hooks project ventrally beyond this surface and are almost exclusively a morbidity affecting maxillary molar teeth. Ramps, on the other hand, are dorsal projections beyond the occlusal surface that affect mandibular molar teeth (CARMALT & RACH, 2003).

THOMASSIAN (2005) defines ramps as hooks that project dorsally, occurring on the caudal molars of the mandible. Because they can't find their opposites, they don't stop growing, developing hooks and ramps. Affected horses suffer a lot of pain when trying to chew, as the projections reach the maxilla - in the case of ramps - and/or the mandible, in the case of hooks (THOMASSIAN, 2005). Hooks can be the result of hereditary occlusal defects or acquired throughout life. The occurrence of hooks prevents the equine from freely developing "side-to-side" chewing movements, as well as rostro-caudal movements, resulting in improper and excessive wear of the premolar and/or molar teeth **(figure 12)**.

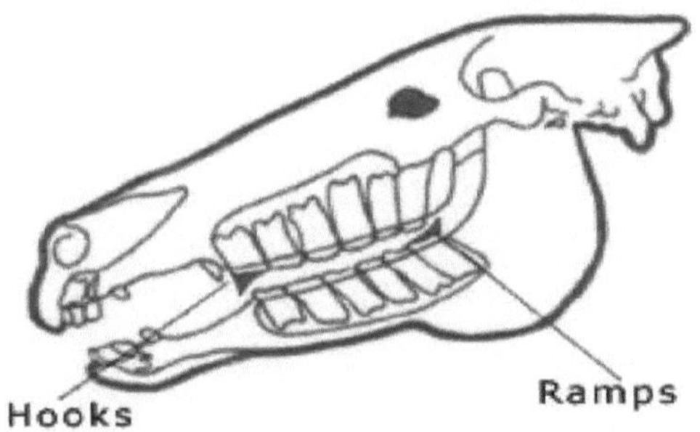

Figura 12 **- Diagram showing ramps**

Source: Adapted from OMURA, (2009)

2.4.9 Wave-like tooth wear

When the teeth erupt at different speeds, this generates a ripple on the occlusal surface in a rostro-caudal direction, commonly referred to by the Americans as "wave mouth". Tooth eruption, in turn, depends on the health of the periodontal membrane, i.e. a healthy membrane promotes good eruption, while an infected membrane promotes delayed tooth eruption. This difference in eruption speed is one of the main causes of waves on the occlusal surface (DIXON & DACRE, 2005).

According to OMURA (2009), this occlusion problem should be treated in stages so that the horse doesn't lose its ability to crush food. If it is very severe, it should not be completely corrected in the first intervention, but with time and good maintenance, it will gradually improve. It consists of reducing the wavy complexes by grinding, while maintaining an appropriate angle of the molar table (OMURA, 2009). **(figure 13)**

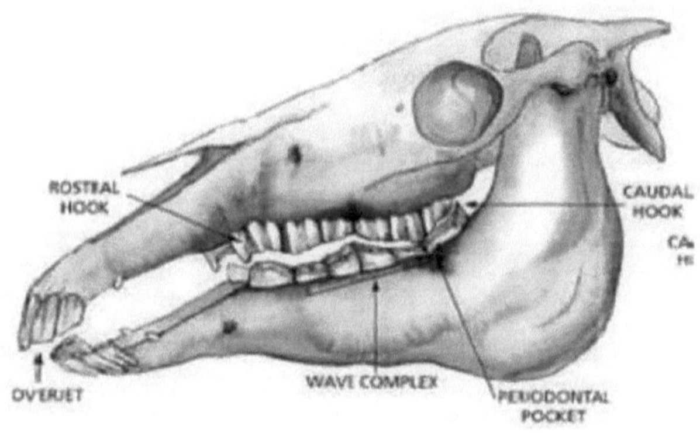

Figura 13 **Oiagram showing tooth wear in waves.**

Source: Adapted from THOMASSIAN, **(2009)**

2.5 FIBER EVALUATION

The process of food digestion in horses begins in the mouth with the grasping of the grass or feed by the lips and incisor teeth. Through chewing (mechanical grinding), the food is reduced to small particles, thus allowing the nutrients to be better utilized. Mouth problems can lead to chewing deficits and the ingestion of poorly ground food, predisposing the horse to develop gastrointestinal disorders (ALVES, 2004).

The mastication test, although very important, has not been fully carried out by most professionals. The ability to chew would be checked by visual observation of masticatory movements concomitant with hearing the sounds during chewing, by extra-oral and intra-oral palpation, inspection of the teeth and feces (ALVES, 2004; DIXON, 2005; EASLEY, 2005).

Attention should be paid to the patient's stool to get an idea of how the food has been processed and digested. Examination of the stool should not reveal the presence of whole grains or forage particles larger than approximately 0.64cm in length (EASLEY, 2005).

Horses with good oral health have better nutrient utilization, reduced risk of intestinal problems and better performance in their athletic and work activities (THOMASSIAN, 2005).

The ingestive behavior of animals is influenced by the structure of the pasture and the heterogeneity of the spatial distribution of vegetation, with the structure of the pasture being the main factor affecting the behavioral variables of animal consumption (EASLEY, 2005).

In extensive management conditions, horses can spend up to 16 hours a day grazing (MEYER,1995).

2.5.1   Pennisetum clandestinum

Pennisetum clandestinum, commonly known as quicuio grass, was brought to Brazil in 1924 and was immediately hailed as being of exceptional quality, having been compared in quality to alfalfa in the early years of its introduction (OTERO, 1946).

It is a perennial grass reaching up to 1 m in height, with thin, hollow, glabrous, tender stems, short internodes; erect or decumbent; the leaves are narrow (5 mm), of varying length (10-30 cm), alternate, invaginating, covered in short, fine hairs, most frequent on the dorsal page. It also has creeping stalks and rhizomes (ANDRADE, 1948).

Quicuio grass has very good digestibility, with indices of 65% for crude protein, 70% for extractives and nitrogen and 60% for crude fiber. It can be used directly as pasture or as raw material for making hay, which is of excellent quality (PUPO, 1985).

In addition to its nutritional quality, another important characteristic of good pasture fodder is its resistance to trampling. This quality has been pointed out by several authors. They also point to the production of good hay as another important characteristic. Next, they pointed out resistance to cold, ease of adaptation to all terrain, rusticity, resistance to drought, ease of sprouting, palatability, resistance to fire, vigor, good carrying capacity, good for cutting, fibrous in drought and suitable for grazing by dairy cows and horses (PUPO, 1985).

2.5.2   Brachiaria humidicola

Brachiaria humidicola is one of the tropical forages widely used to feed service horses in the cerrado areas of Central Brazil, where it is practically the only forage option apart from native pastures (MEYER, 1995).

It is a perennial grass from the African continent, where it occurs in relatively humid areas. Adapted to the climate and soil conditions of the Cerrado, it grows well in regions with weak soils and high acidity, and is easily propagated by seeds and seedlings. However, the use of pastures of this species for horses, in relation to its desirable agronomic characteristics, is generally not well accepted. The horses that use it show delayed development, low work performance, as well as health problems and metabolic disorders. Intoxication, lameness, indisposition, tiredness, weight loss, fractures and even death often occur (SILVA, 2004).

The main causes of these problems lie in the low quality of the fodder, especially low protein and mineral content, high fiber content and high concentrations of toxic principles (oxalates). Protein deficits in animals' diets usually interfere with their development and performance (MEYER, 1995).

Brachiaria humidicola grass has crude protein = 6.73, neutral detergent fiber = 67.8; dry matter = 33.80 (SILVA, 2004)

3 METHODOLOGICAL PROCEDURE

A literature search was carried out, looking at information on the subject in scientific articles, specialized magazines, books and reputable websites with scientific characteristics.

A descriptive, longitudinal field study was carried out in order to collect data that can characterize the objectives set out in the study to be investigated. The research will be quantitative in nature.

Data was collected through dental prophylaxis applied to 30 horses between the ages of four and nineteen, nine males and twenty-one females with an average body weight of 350kg and a body score of 3.

The horses belonged to two properties, one located in the municipality of Linhares and the other in Colatina, Espirito Santo. The animals were used for routine work on the properties for ten hours a day. They had complete dental arches, with excessive enamel tips, waves, steps, wolf teeth, flattening and swallow tails, but no history of dietary changes or dental treatment. The diet consisted of *Brachiaria humidicola* and Quicuio grass *(Pennisetum clandestinum)*.

The experimental period was divided into two phases. In the first, the animals were occlusally adjusted, fecal samples were taken from the rectal ampulla, without the use of lubricants, only with the aid of water and procedural gloves, so as not to alter the final drying, in the amount of 200 grams and the dental disorders found were noted.

The samples were identified according to the numbering of the animals, weighed and stored in Kraft paper bags, processed in a drying oven at 60°c and kept for 72 hours in the university's chemistry laboratory. After drying, the samples were weighed and sieved to separate the fibers and measured with a millimeter ruler, noting the size of the largest and smallest fibers found.

The second phase began seven to fifteen days after the first and consisted of a new collection of feces, processing and measurement of fecal fibers.

During dental treatment, the animals underwent a complete clinical examination before and after each procedure. After fasting for 12 hours, the animals were weighed using a tape for measuring the thoracic perimeter of horses, and sedation was carried out using Detomidine Hydrochloride (0.02mg/kg) and, when necessary, Butorphanol Tartrate (1ml/UA) intravenously. Repeats of Detomidine Hydrochloride were given at a dose of one third of the animal's initial dose, administered according to the duration of the dental treatment. With the animal sedated and restrained in the trunk, the oral cavity was rinsed with running water to remove any dirt and the incisor teeth were inspected (claws, middle and corners). After the examination, a Hausmmam-type mouth opener was used to inspect the oral cavity, with a spotlight and a dental mirror for detailed visual inspection of the other dental elements (premolars and molars). Dental prophylaxis consisted of corrective wear of the excessive tips of tooth enamel and the other disorders found. The materials used for corrective wear were: electric rasps and manual rasps.

When the wolf tooth was extracted, an anesthetic block was applied to the hard palate with Lidocaine Hydrochloride 2.5 ml per tooth, divided between the rostral and caudal folds of the tooth, The tooth elevator **(figure 15)** was then used to elevate the gums and perform a syndesmotomy of the tooth, with the aid of a dolphin head appliance **(figure 14)**, bucco-lingual movements were performed to break the dental ligaments and remove the tooth.

During the experimental period, food samples of 200 grams were collected at random from the animals' common feeding area and stored in plastic Kraft paper bags to be dried at 60 °C for 72 hours to assess the fiber composition.

The results will be presented in the form of graphs and tables to determine the conclusion of this research.

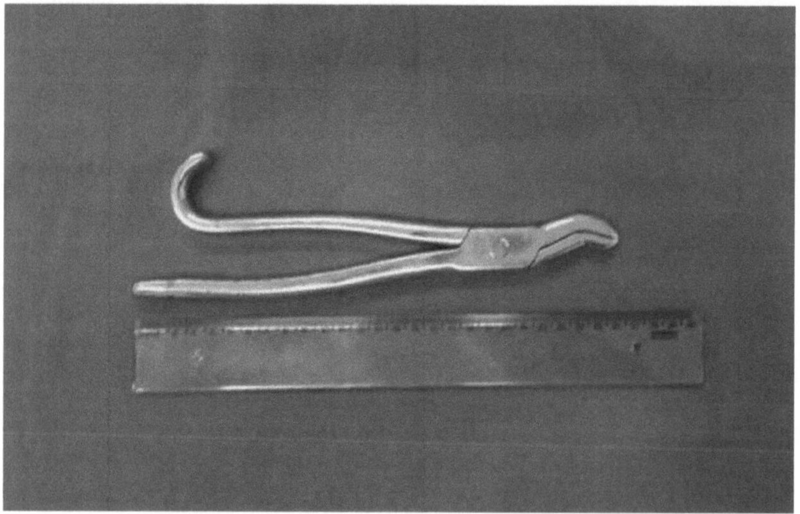

Figure 14 - Dolphin head apothecary.

Source: Personal archive.

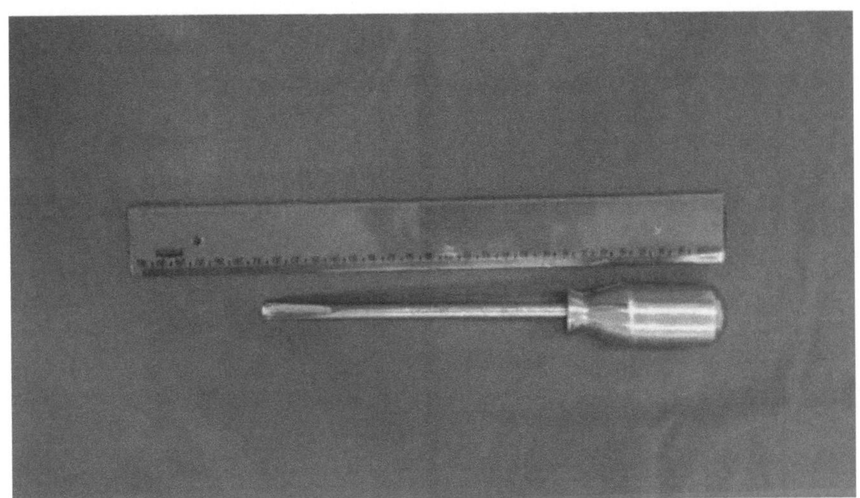

Figure 15 - Tooth elevator.

Source: Personal archive

4 RESULTS AND DISCUSSION

From the analysis and discussion of the selected bibliographic material, it was possible to see that the dental morphology of horses can undergo various and severe alterations over the course of the animal's life, which can be due to the animal's own nature - chronology of ageing - or consequent to pathologies, accidents or even failures in their daily management, which cannot be neglected.

After occlusal adjustment in animals that had never undergone dental treatment, fecal fibers decreased by an average of 0.58 cm, as shown in Table 1. These results were lower than those reported by BOTELHO *et al.* (2007) of 0.63 cm, but they prove the effectiveness of biannual occlusal adjustment in horses.

Table 1 - Comparative table of the first and second phases of fecal fiber collection in the 30 horses evaluated at intervals of seven to fifteen days, with the maximum and minimum sizes found in each fecal sample.

ANIMAL	SIZE FIBER/CM 1ST COLLECTION	SIZE FIBER/CM 2ND COLLECTION
01	3cm /7cm	2cm /5cm
02	3cm/5cm	2cm/3cm
03	3cm/7cm	2cm/4cm
04	7cm/10cm	4cm/6cm
05	3cm	2cm
06	7cm/12cm	4cm/7cm
07	2cm	1,5cm

08	1,5cm	1cm
09	1cm	0,7cm
10	3cm	2,5cm
11	2cm/3cm	2cm
12	0.6cm /1cm	0,6cm
13	2cm	1cm
14	4cm	2,5cm
15	2cm	1cm
16	1cm	1cm
17	2cm	1,5cm
18	2cm/3cm	2cm
19	0.7cm/2cm	0.7cm/1cm
20	2cm	3cm
21	5cm/7cm	2cm
22	2cm	1cm
23	2cm	1,5cm
24	5cm	4cm
25	4cm	3cm
26	1cm	1cm
27	6cm	4cm
28	3cm	2,5cm
29	2cm/3cm	2,5cm
30	4cm	3,5cm
Average	**3,13 cm**	**2.55 cm**

Average 0.58 cm

total

Source: Properties in Linhares and Colatina - ES

To obtain the final result, an average calculation was made between the largest

and smallest fiber found in each sample, then the average of the first collection,

before dental prophylaxis, was made, adding all the values and dividing by the total of 30 animals, finding the group average of 3.13 cm of fibers present in the feces. The same procedure was carried out to obtain the average of the second collection, 7 to 15 days after dental prophylaxis, and the average value of 2.55 cm of fibers was found, arriving at a final difference of 0.58 cm from the first to the second sample.

DIXON ET AL (2011) cited a study carried out by BRIGHAM & DUNCANSON in 2000 in which they analyzed the premolars and molars of 50 slaughterhouse equine skulls and found the following frequencies: 20% of anomalous diastemas, 26% with steps, 56% with excessive tooth enamel tips, 20% with no tooth elements, 8% with waves and 12% with cavities. EASLEY ET AL (2011) reported that the main dental wear alterations are: steps, hooks, waves, excessive transverse ridges and "shear mouth".

As shown in Table 2, the main dental alterations found in the 30 horses were: excessive tips of tooth enamel or PEED (100%), ramp (13.33%), flattening (10%), rostral hook (20%), dovetail (23.33%), ulcer (23.33%), wolf tooth (20%) and wave (6.66%). Shown in Graph 1 below.

Table 2 - Affections found in the 30 horses evaluated in the properties of Linhares and Colatina - ES, aged between four and nineteen years.

Animal	PEED	Hook	Wolf's tooth	Ulcer	Andorin tail ha	Flattening	Ramp	Wave
01	x	211	205		103/203			
02	x							
03	x			x	103/203			

04	x			x	103/203	109	x	x
05	x							
06	x	Rostr albilateral		x	103/203			
07	x					208		
08	x							
09	x						x	
10	x		105/205					
11	x							x
12	x							
13	x						x	
14	x	406		x				
15	x		105					
16	x							
17	x							
18	x	406		x			x	
19	x							
20	x		105/205					
21	x	311		x	103/203	309		
22	x							
23	x		105/205					
24	x							
25	x	Rostr al /bilateral		x	103/203			
26	x							
27	x							
28	x		105/205					

29	x							
30	x			103/203				

Source: Properties in Linhares and Colatina - ES

Graph 1 - Frequency, in percentages, of the main alterations found in 30 horses examined at the properties in Linhares and Colatina - ES

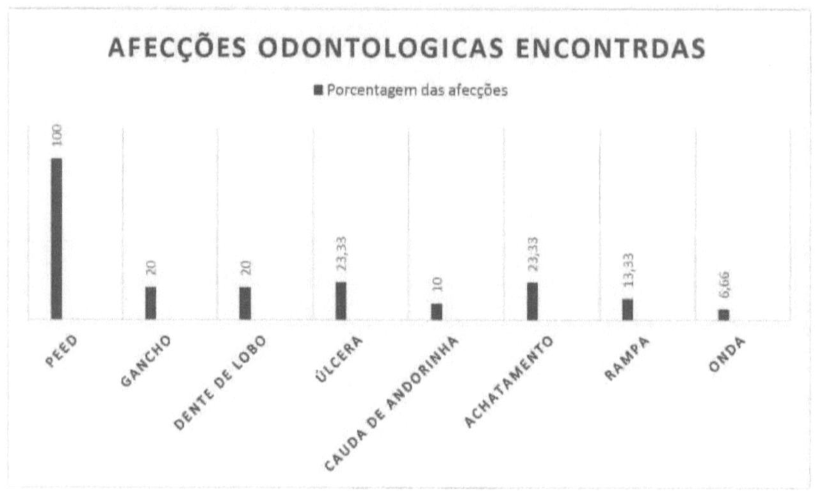

Source: Properties in Linhares and Colatina - ES

According to Table 2, we can see that the dental disorders are present in association with each other, which creates greater discomfort for the animal, altering the biomechanics of mastication and resulting in poorer crushing of the food. In animals with more than one dental disorder, it was possible to see greater alterations in the sizes and quantities of the fecal fibers analyzed. Dental alterations change according to the animal's age and diet.

CONCLUSION

As has been discussed throughout this work, the oral cavity of horses is usually the site of various alterations that occur mainly in the teeth and periodontium.

It is therefore necessary to have a good knowledge of the structure and anatomy of the equine oral cavity, the physiology of chewing, the main methods of assessing the oral cavity, the main signs of dental alterations and the most frequently encountered pathologies. It is also essential to master the main instruments and therapeutic methods used to solve them.

The main objective of the work was to show the importance of occlusal adjustment in horses through the evaluation and measurement of fecal fibers, bearing in mind that dental prophylaxis carried out biannually generates masticatory comfort in the animal, improving the grinding of ingested food, generating an improvement in digestibility, which results in lower fecal fibers.

Measuring fecal fibers is a rarely used method for assessing oral health, due to the time it takes to process the samples, but it would be extremely important in helping to diagnose previous illnesses in horses.

REFERENCES

ALVES, G., PAGLIOSA, G., SANTOS, J. (2004). *Mini-course in equine dentistry. VI CongressAlves*, G.E.S. 2004. **Dentistry as part of gastroenterology**: health and digestibility. p. 7-22. In: Alves, G.E.S., Pagliosa, G.M., Santos, J.A.M. (ed.) *Congresso Brasileiro de Cirurgia e Anestesia Veterinària - Mini Curso De Odontologia Equina*, 6. Jaguariuna College, Indaiatuba.

ANDRADE, B. M., 1948 - Formation and Treatment of Pastures. S. I. A. Ministry of Agriculture, Rio de Janeiro, Brazil.

BAKER, G.J. **Dental physiology**. In: EASLEY, K.J.; BAKER, G.J. *Equine dentistry*. London: W.B. Saunders, 2002. p.29-34.

BOTELHO, D.L.M.; CESAR, J.A. W.; FILADELPHO, A.L. Equine Odontology. **Electronic Scientific Journal of Veterinary Medicine**. Year IV, n.8, 2007. *Brazilian Journal of Veterinary Surgery and Anesthesiology, Indaiatuba, Sao Paulo, Brazil*. Accessed

BREDER, A. **UNIVERTIX VETERINARY MEDICINE BLOG**.

Available at:

<http://equipeveterinariafv2010.blogspot.com.br/2010/08/odontologia-equina.html>. Accessed on November 13, 2014.

CARMALT, J.; RACH, D. **Equine Dentistry** - Moving into the 21st Century.

Large Animal Veterinary Rounds, v. 3, n. 5, mai/2003

CARNEIRO, J; JUNQUEIRA, L. C. **Histologia bàsica**. 8 ed. Rio de Janeiro: Guanabara Koogan, 1995.

DACRE, I. **Physiology of mastication**. *Focus meeting, Indianopolis, USA.* 2006. Available at:< *www.ivis.org/proceedings/aaepfocus/2006/itdacre1.pdf>*. *Accessed* on July 29, 2014.

DACRE, I.; DIXON, P.M. A review of equine dental disorders. *The Veterinary Journal,* 2005.

DART, A.J.; PASCOE, R.R.**Treatment of abilateral mandibular fracture in a mare using an intraoral acrylic splint**. Aust. Vet.1987.

DIXON et al. Equine dental disease Part 2: a long-term study of 400 cases: disorders of development and eruption and variations in position of the cheek teeth. *Equine veterinary journal.* 1999.

DIXON, P.M. Dental anatomy. In G.J. Baker & J. Easley (eds.), *Equine dentistry*. 1999. W.B. Saunders Company.

DIXON, P.M; DU TOIT, N. Common dental disorders in the donkey.

Equine Veterinary Education, v.24, n.1, p.45-51, 2012. Available at: *<http://www.equalli.com.br/upload/textos/pdf/prt/64.pdf>*. Accessed on July 29, 2014.

EASKEY, K.J. Equine dental development and anatomy. In: ANNUAL CONVENTION OF THE AMERICAN ASSOCIATION OF EQUINE PRACTITIONERS,42.,1996,Phoenix, Arizona. **Proceedings**...,1996

EASKEY, K.J. Equine dental development and anatomy. In: ANNUAL CONVENTION OF THE AMERICAN ASSOCIATION OF EQUINE PRACTITIONERS,42.,1996,Denver, CO. **Proceedings**..., 2004

FOSTER, D.L. (2008). Aging guidelines. In J.A. Orsini & T.J. Divers (eds.). *Equine Emergencies: treatment and procedures.* 3 ed. (pp.173176). W. B. Saunders Company.

FRAPE, D. **Equine nutrition & feeding**. 3.ed. Sâo Paulo: Roca, 2008.

GORREL, C. (1997). Equine dentistry: evolution and structure. *Equine veterinary journal*.

KRELING, K. *Horses' teeth and their problems: prevention, recognition and treatment.* 2 ed. Germany: Cadmos, 2003.

LOWDER,Q. M.; MUELLER, P.O.E. Dental embryology, anatomy, development and aging. **Veterinary Clinics of Noth America - Equine Practice**, v. 14, 1998.

MANSO, C.; SAN ROMAN, F. Historia clinica y exploración da la cavidad oral. *Equinus*, 2 ed. 2002.

MEYER, H. **Feeding horses**. 2.ed. Sâo Paulo: Varela, 1995.

OMURA, C. M. Dentes e Companhia - Equine Odontology. *http://equinocompleto.com.sapo.pt/w004.htm.* 31 Mar 2009. Accessed on Nov. 10, 2014.

OTERO, J. R., 1946 - O Capim Kikuyù, S. D. A. - 310, 2nd ed. Minist. Agr., Rio de Janeiro.

PUPO, N. I. H. Manual de pastagens e forrageiras. Campinas: Instituto Campineiro de Ensino Agrìcola, 1985

RALSTON, S.L.; FOSTER, D.L.; DIVERS, T.; HINTZ, H.F. Effect of dental correction on feed digestibility in horses. **Equine Veterinary Journal**. n.33, v.4, 2001.

SILVA et al. Estimating the age of horses through dental examination. *Revista portuguesa de ciências veterinàrias*, 2003.

SILVA, L.A.C. et al. Grazing behavior and food preference of Pantanal horses used in the daily management of Pantanal cattle. In: ANNUAL MEETING OF THE BRAZILIAN SOCIETY OF ZOOTECHNICS, 41, 2004, Campo Grande. Proceedings... Campo Grande-MS: EMBRAPA, 2004.

SMITH, B. P. **Large animal internal medicine**, 3 ed. Barueri, SP: Manole, 2006.

SMOLDERS, E.A.A.; STEG, A.; HINDLE, V.A. Organic matter digestibility in horses and its prediction. *J. Agric. Sci.*, v.38, 1990.

SOUZA, L.M.P. **Equine dentistry**. 2009. Available at: *<http://www.informativoequinos.com.br/Vet.%20odontologia.htm>*. Accessed on Nov. 10, 2014.

THOMASSIAN, A. **Equine diseases**. 4 ed. Sâo Paulo: Livraria Varela, 2005.

VAN SOEST, P.J. Development of a comprehensive system of feed analyses and its application to forages. *J. Anim. Sci.*,1967.

ANNEX

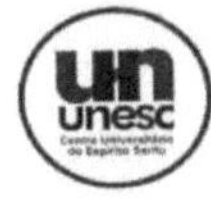

CENTRO UNIVERSITÁRIO DO ESPÍRITO SANTO

-UNESC-

CEUA - CONSUBSTANTIATED Opinion

RESEARCH PROJECT DATA

Research title: Effectiveness of dental prophylaxis in horses in terms of fecal fiber evaluation.

Researcher: Prof. Diogo Almeida Rondon

Knowledge Area (CNPq): Veterinary Medicine- 50502050- Animal Health

Proposing Institution: Centro Universitário do Espirilo Santo

OPINION DATA

Opinion Number: 246574

Reporting date: 02/05/2015

Project presentation: The study addresses the quality of chewing and digested fibers during dental prophylaxis in horses. This is a qualitative study.

Research objective: To evaluate the effectiveness of the procedure on digestibility and chewing quality.

Assessment of Risks and Benefits: The benefits are inherent to the knowledge to be covered and the risks are related to the practical procedure described in the study methodology.

Comments and Considerations on the Research: The anesthetic and clinical protocols are in accordance with the ethical and biosafety principles of the methodology described.

Considerations regarding the Terms of Mandatory Submission: All the forms have been sent and filled in all the fields that identify the study.

Recommendations: Carry out the methodology proposed in the study.

Conclusions or Outstanding Issues and List of Inadequacies: According to the research methodology presented, there are no outstanding issues.

Opinion Status: APPROVED

COLATINA, 02 de maio de 2015

YOLANDA CHRISTINA DE SOUSA LOYOLA

(Coordenador)

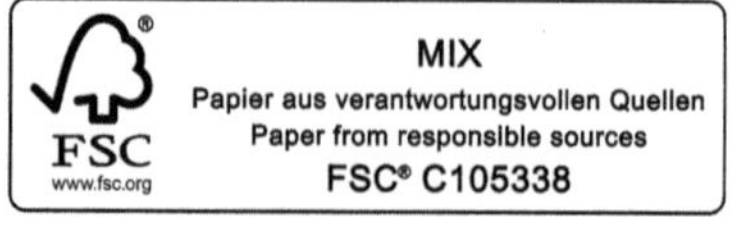

Printed by Books on Demand GmbH, Norderstedt / Germany